PELVIC FLOOR MANUAL FOR EXERCISES

A STEP BY STEP EXCERCISING MOVES FOR PELVIC FLOOR

CALEB THIESFIELD

Table of Contents

CHAPTER ONE

MOVES THAT BENEFIT THE PELVIC FLOOR

Anyone and Everyone Can Benefit from Pelvic Floor Exercises

Sneezing, laughing, and coughing can all cause you to pee a little. You're not the only one. Pelvic floor disorders are common and can strike anyone at any time.

In a nutshell? Strengthening your pelvic floor muscles and reducing the severity of pelvic organ prolapse symptoms can both be achieved by including specific exercises (also known as "pelvic floor muscle training").

Here's a simple explanation of the pelvic floor, including what it is, what it does, where to look for it, and when to seek professional help. Plus, there are five exercises that you can begin immediately to strengthen your pelvic floor!

It is made up of a network of muscles and tendons and ligaments. Specifically, the bones at the bottom of your pelvis are attached by these soft tissues.

Peripheral organs include the urethra (urethrae), bladder (bladder), rectum (rectum). Uterus, cervix, and vagina comprise the pelvic floor in women who have them.

Marcy Crouch, PT, DPT, WCS, a board-certified clinical specialist in women's health, recommends picturing the pelvic floor muscles as a hammock or basket at the bottom of the pelvis.

To stop gas or urine or pucker your anal opening, the pelvic floor has to be engaged or contracted, which causes a lifting motion toward the head.

The muscles and tissues of the pelvic floor are attached to the pelvis by the pelvic floor muscles and tissues.

Pelvic floor functions include what?

A person's daily activities depend heavily on the muscles of the pelvic floor. Urinary, genital, anus, and vaginal organs are all supported by the bladder and the urethra.

In addition to arousal and orgasm, the pelvic floor muscles play an important role in sexual health and function.

When you're walking or standing, they help keep your hips and back in place.

Vaginal birth and pregnancy-related muscle weakness can lead to a variety of problems, from mild discomfort and pain to pelvic organ prolapse.

Pelvic floor dysfunction can occur for a variety of reasons, not just during pregnancy or childbirth. This condition can also be triggered by the onset of menopause, a history of heavy lifting or prolonged sitting, sexual abuse, or other conditions that put pressure on the abdomen.

Pelvic floor disorders (PFD) can also be exacerbated by certain habits, symptoms, or conditions, such as irritable bowel syndrome, interstitial cystitis, and habitual bowel movement avoidance or restriction.

The urethra, bladder, rectum, and other pelvic organs are supported by the pelvic floor muscles. Having a uterus, cervix and vagina means that the pelvic floor also supports these organs.

Many people associate Kegels and the pelvic floor with a vagina and, more specifically, pregnancy when they think of these terms.

In fact, these muscles are present in both men and women. The muscles of the pelvic floor support the bladder and bowel in men who have a penis, preventing stool and urine leakage.

They also aid in the maintenance of sexual health,

including the ability to feel and perform sexually.

Chronic prostatitis, pudendal neuralgia, genitofemoral neuralgia, and hypertonicity are among the most common diagnoses of pelvic floor disorders in men.

What is the best method for locating the muscles of the pelvic floor?

Finding the pelvic floor is as simple as slowing or stopping urine flow while using the restroom. After a few successful attempts, you've discovered your pelvic floor.

CHAPTER TWO

Crouch suggests the following as an additional method of energizing the muscles of the pelvic floor:

Kneel on the floor with your feet flat on the floor. Inhale.

Relax your lower abdominal muscles and the muscles around the urethra as if you're trying to stop gas or urine from leaking out of your body. For those with vaginas, lifting or squeezing the muscles around the vagina can also be an important part of their workout.

Hold for a few seconds, and then let go of it all. You should feel the muscles in your pelvic floor relax and fall.

While standing, imagine that you need to urinate but don't want to. This will help you locate the pelvic floor muscles.

Trying to keep it in will likely result in rectus and anus squeezing. If you feel a tugging sensation at your anus, the muscles in your pelvic floor should be activated.

It's critical to keep in mind that the muscles of the pelvic floor extend all the way to your pubic bone. It's not getting a full contraction if you're only contracting the muscles that control urine flow but not the rectal muscles.

Engage both the muscles that stop gas and the muscles that stop urine simultaneously for the most effective contraction. Pelvic floor muscle engagement can also be improved by simultaneously activating the transversus abdominis and obliques.

Engaging the pelvic floor muscles, on the other hand, may help to strengthen the abdominal contraction.

This is especially true if you're an active person or if you're trying to build functional core strength.

Learning how to relax these muscles is just as important for proper pelvic floor function as learning how to hold them in place. Do a self-check now and then to see if you're always feeling the contraction of these muscles, even just a little bit.

Consider the muscles of your pelvic floor as an elevator. Take note of where the elevator has come to a halt when you're sitting at your desk or standing to do the dishes. Is it on the first or second level? What floor are you on? At the tenth, or even further back?

Excessive muscle tension in these areas can lead to pain if

you don't learn to let the elevator rest at the bottom.

Many methods exist for locating the pelvic floor muscles, such as stopping the flow of urine and preventing gas from exiting the body. It's critical to master the art of both contracting and relaxing these muscle groups simultaneously.

How common is pelvic floor dysfunction?

A weak or malfunctioning pelvic floor causes pelvic floor disorders when the pelvic floor muscles are unable to adequately support the pelvic organs.

Painful sex may be a sign of a urinary or fecal leak, urgency urinary incontinence, an overactive bladder, or pelvic organ prolapse.

Pelvic floor disorders are difficult to estimate because awareness of their symptoms and conditions is low. People who identify as female are more likely to avoid treatment for pelvic floor dysfunction because they believe it's a normal part of childbirth or aging.

It is estimated that one in four women suffer from pelvic floor disorders, and that number doubles by the time women reach their 80th birthdays. According to some studies, about half of pregnant women are affected by PFD.

Furthermore, researchers predict that the number of women affected by PFD will rise by 70% by the year 2050 as a result of health trends such as rising BMI and chronic constipation.

People with a penis don't usually think they're affected by PFD, but the prevalence of such conditions in men is estimated to be around 16 percent.

Pelvic floor dysfunction presents with the following symptoms:

a feeling of fullness or pressure in the lower abdomen

• frequent urination or urination that is painful

• Leakage of urine

• incontinence of the bladder

pain in the lower back

Constipation,bowel obstructions, or leaking stools

• inability to eliminate waste from the body

Anxiety and/or discomfort during a sexual encounter

• discomfort in the genitals or pelvic region

spasms of the pelvic muscles

Many people with PFD can find relief from pain and embarrassment by using nonsurgical methods to treat the condition. The first step is usually to see a pelvic floor physical therapy specialist.

Do I have an inflexible pelvic floor?

If you have a long-term problem with your pelvic floor, it could be caused by either hypotonic and hypertonic muscle groups (pelvic floor muscles that are too tight or overactive) Relaxing pelvic floor dysfunction and nonrelaxing pelvic floor dysfunction are sometimes referred to as two separate conditions.

Both hypotonic and hypertonic issues can occur on a continuum with pelvic floor dysfunction. Inactive muscles are frequently blamed for pelvic floor issues, which is why many people are shocked to learn the opposite is true.

However, not everyone should engage in Kegel exercises.

Skeletal muscle constitutes the pelvic floor. "That means it can be injured, weak, or traumatized in the same way as any other muscle in your body," explains Crouch. A calf muscle spasm, for example, can cause it to become "tight" or chronically contracted.

Doing Kegels, according to Crouch, can exacerbate symptoms such as cramping, leaking urine, constipation, and even sexual dysfunction if the muscles are already tight. A hypertonic pelvic floor should be avoided until a pelvic floor physical therapist is consulted.

Strengthening one's pelvic floor has a number of advantages.

After a full contraction of the rectus abdominis muscle, the pelvic floor should be able to fully relax. The bladder, bowels, and uterus can all be better supported by strengthening the pelvic floor.

In addition, it can aid in the control of the bladder and bowels.

Improved pelvic floor function has also been found to improve quality of life, according to researchers.

The symptoms of pelvic floor prolapse, such as urinary leakage, incontinence, pelvic pressure, and lower back pain, can all be alleviated by strengthening the pelvic floor muscles.

Better sex may also result from a program to strengthen the pelvic floor.

According to a few studies, male sexual function and pelvic floor function may be linked. Pelvic floor physical therapy, in particular, has been shown to improve erectile dysfunction and ejaculation issues, according to researchers.

To further enhance sexual sensation and function, some people with a vagina benefit from regularly squeezing or contracting the pelvic floor muscles.

Last but not least, the American Urological Association

recommends pelvic floor muscle training as a way to manage an overactive bladder.

It is hoped that this treatment will reduce incontinence by inhibiting uncontrolled bladder contractions.

Pelvic floor strengthening exercises

The pelvic floor can be activated at any time and in any place. The pelvic floor muscles can also be strengthened and targeted through specific exercises.

For those with hypotonic pelvic floor muscles, one way to design a program is to categorize the exercises according to their level of activity.

In the words of Crouch, hypotonic means that you have low pelvic floor tone and that you need to improve your endurance and strength.

Hypotonic pelvic floor muscle strengthening exercises

Crouch suggests the following three exercises to treat hypotonicity of the pelvic floor:

In a matter of seconds, perform Kegels.

According to Crouch, a quick flick In order to stop leaks when sneezing or coughing, Kegel requires quick contractions of the pelvic floor muscles.

To begin, lie on your back with your knees bent and your feet flat on the ground. Sit or stand while doing this exercise as you get more comfortable with it.

Find your pelvic muscles by following the aforementioned guidelines.

When you exhale, pull your navel toward your spine and quickly contract and release your pelvic floor muscles. 3. Aim for a one-second contraction and release.

Breathe normally throughout the entire process.

Afterwards, take a 10-second break and repeat the quick flick 10 times. Do two to three sets.

CHAPTER THREE

Slides on the heel

Pelvic floor contractions are aided by heel slides, which also work the deep abdominal muscles.

Lie on your stomach, knees bent, and pelvis neutral on the floor to begin.

Allow your ribs to naturally compress by inhaling into your

rib cage and then exhaling through your mouth.

Draw your pelvic floor up, lock in your core, and slide your right heel away from you in a counter-clockwise direction. If you lose your connection to your deep core, you've gone too far, and you should stop.

Inhale and return your leg to the starting position after you've found the bottom position.

Repeat.

Do a total of 10 slides on each side before switching to the next leg.

I'm on the move! (also called toe taps)

The marching exercise, like heel slides, improves core stability and stimulates contractions of the pelvic floor.

Lie on your stomach, knees bent, and pelvis neutral on the floor to begin.

When you exhale, allow your ribs to naturally compress as you inhale into them.

. Lift your pelvic floor and tighten your abdominal muscles.

Lift one leg to a tabletop position and slowly lower it back down.

Slowly bring this leg back to the starting position..

Repeat the movement with each leg, switching them out. You shouldn't feel any discomfort in your lower back at all. To get the most benefit from this exercise, make sure your deep core stays engaged the entire time.

Do this for 12–20 times, alternating legs.

exercises for pelvic floor muscles that are overly tight and tense

Hypertonic exercises may help someone with a short or tight pelvic floor relax and lengthen.

So that muscle contractions can be more effective, Crouch

recommends releasing and lengthening the hypertonic muscle groups. Lengthening and strengthening go hand in hand, she explains, because "we have to make sure the muscle can do what we need it to do."

She suggests the following two exercises to help you get started:

Pose your baby in a happy mood.

When you want to stretch and release your pelvic floor, the

Happy Baby Pose is a great addition.

Start by bending your knees and lying on the floor.
Make a 90-degree angle with your knees and place your feet with the soles facing up.

The outside or inside of your feet can be grabbed and held.

In other words, you want your knees to be about an inch or two wider than your chest. Then, raise your feet so that they are level with your elbows.

Your ankles should be above your knees at all times.

 Push your feet into your hands and flex your heels. Allow yourself several breaths or a gentle rocking motion in this position.

breathing with the diaphragm
This method of breathing uses the diaphragm in conjunction with the pelvic floor to promote a healthy relationship between the two muscles. As a bonus, it's an excellent way to relieve stress.

CHAPTER FOUR

Practice progressive relaxation for a few seconds. Take time to relax your muscles.

Put one hand on your stomach and the other on your chest once you've calmed down.

The stomach should expand as you inhale through your nose, but your chest should remain relatively still. 4. Finally, inhale and exhale slowly for 2–3 seconds, then repeat.

After a few repetitions of this exercise, switch hands and hold each one on the chest and stomach.

Lunges and squats are also recommended by Crouch as part of a pelvic floor exercise program. Adding in pelvic floor strengthening exercises such as lunging and Swiss ball squats, she says, can be a simple way to get started.

Think about contracting the pelvic floor before descending into a lunge or squat, and then re-engaging at the bottom and contracting again as you rise to standing.

How often should you see a doctor?

Adding daily pelvic floor exercises to one's regimen is an easy way to keep one's pelvic floor muscles strong and healthy.

A doctor or therapist trained in pelvic floor issues may be necessary for some people, however. In particular, if you're dealing with bowel or bladder control issues, this is a must.

Here are a few warning signs that it's time to see a doctor.

- peeing or pooping on the floor

- difficulty urinating or bowel movements

- Pelvic pain or discomfort

- noticing or experiencing a bulge in the vagina or anus

- Urinary incontinence

- incontinence

- inability to completely empty the bladder or bowels

To be on the safe side, call your doctor even if your symptoms seem mild. Getting the right care for your condition can make you feel better and protect the pelvic floor from further damage.

The nitty-gritty

You can strengthen your pelvic floor muscles and improve your overall health by including them in your daily routine. Keep in mind the importance of proper form and function, as well as the importance of activating the muscles during each exercise.

It's best to seek the advice of an expert in pelvic floor physical therapy if you're new to these exercises or just need some extra guidance. They are able to make specific recommendations for exercises and ensure that you are performing them correctly.

A doctor's appointment should be made as soon as possible if your symptoms are interfering

with your daily activities or
seem to be getting worse.

THE END

www.ingramcontent.com/pod-product-compliance
Lightning Source LLC
Chambersburg PA
CBHW061644130726
47996CB00003B/1449